The year's Lippincott Pocket Medicine Handbook for Nurses

A Comprehensive, Invaluable Resource for Nurses Worldwide

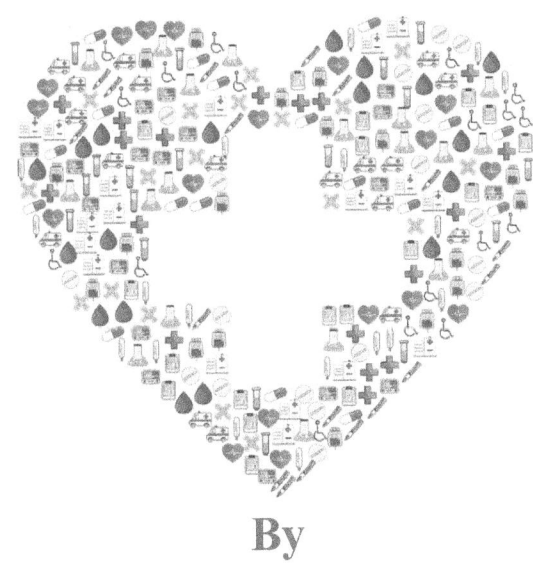

By

Sarah Evans

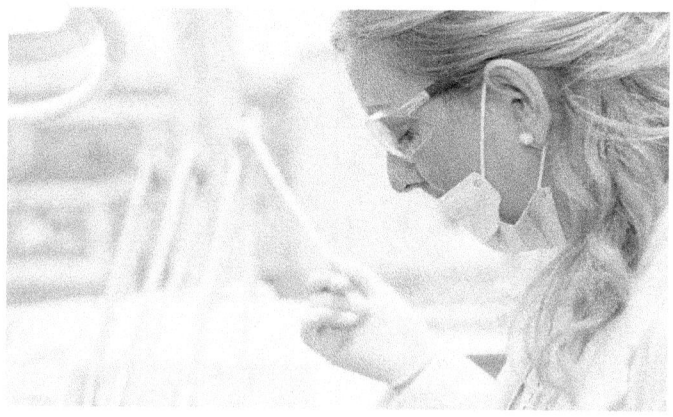

Table of content

Introduction

In the quick developing scene of current medical services, where each choice can be basic and each second counts, attendants stand as the bleeding edge champions of patient consideration.

In this unique climate, the requirement for dependable, directionally advanced handbooks has never been more urgent.

This presentation investigates the meaning of such assets, with a specific spotlight on the renowned genealogy of the Lippincott Pocket Medication Handbooks and their basic job in molding nursing greatness.

A Short History of Lippincott Pocket Medication Handbooks:

For a really long time, Lippincott Pocket Medication Handbooks have been inseparable from greatness in nursing care and schooling.

With every release, these smaller yet extensive aides have filled in as confided in allies for medical caretakers, offering succinct, proof based data readily available. As we commend this tradition of greatness, we perceive the significant effect these handbooks have had on forming the training and instruction of nursing experts around the world.

The High-Stakes, Quick moving Climate of Present day Medical services:

In the present medical services scene, medical attendants wind up exploring a high-stakes, quick moving climate where the requests are tenacious and a lot is on the line.

From shuffling numerous patients to pursuing basic choices like a flash, attendants are entrusted with guaranteeing patient wellbeing and care quality in the midst of steadily expanding difficulties.

This part dives into the intricacies of current medical services and the interesting tensions looked by nursing experts on the cutting edges of patient consideration.

How the Lippincott Pocket Medication Handbook for Attendants Engages Nursing Experts:

In the midst of the turmoil of the medical services climate, the Lippincott Pocket Medication Handbook for Attendants arises as a priceless asset, enabling nursing experts with the information and certainty expected to explore different clinical situations.

 Whether in emergency clinics, centers, long haul care offices, or past, this handbook fills in as a reference point of direction, furnishing medical attendants with fundamental data on prescriptions, techniques, evaluations, and mediations.

Through its easy to understand arrangement and proof based content, this handbook empowers medical caretakers to convey ideal consideration, maintain patient wellbeing, and succeed in their work, guaranteeing that they stay at the bleeding edge of medical services greatness.

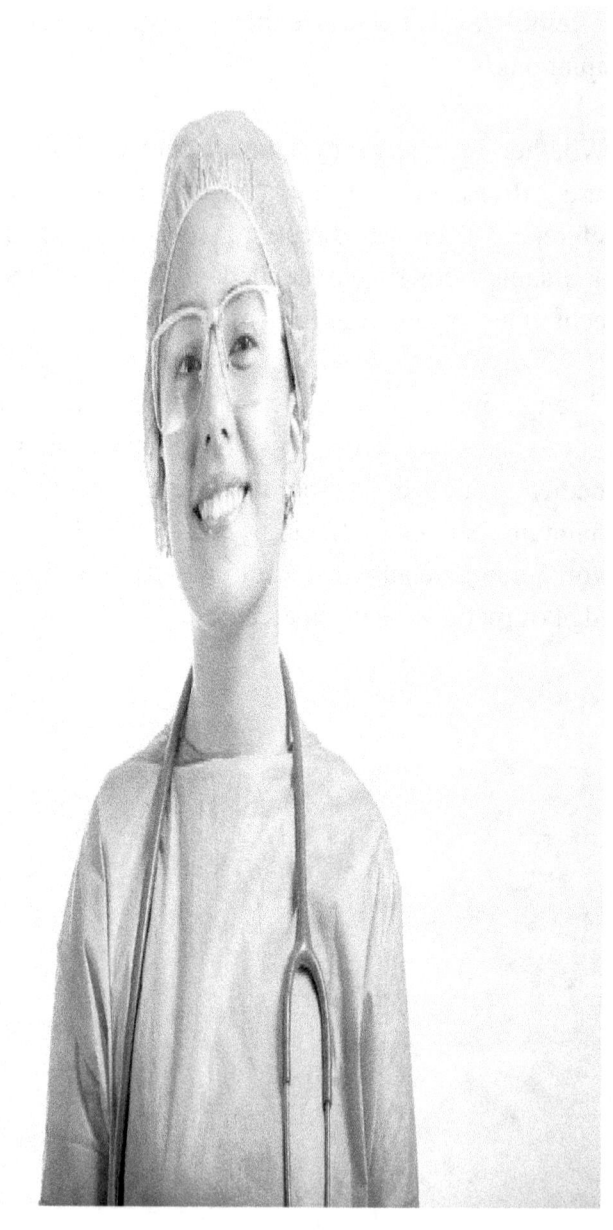

Section One: Quick Facts

In this part, we'll give a speedy reference manual for the vital updates and changes introduced in the current year's Pocket Medication Handbook.

We'll sum up significant modifications across key segments and parts, present new benefactors and master critiques, and deal with a fast manual for exploring the handbook's center areas and exceptional elements.

Synopsis of Significant Updates, Corrections, and Enhancements:

The current year's release of the Pocket Medication Handbook integrates a few huge updates and corrections to guarantee it stays a complete and dependable asset for nursing experts. A portion of the significant updates include:

1. Extended Medication Information: Refreshed drug measurements, organization rules, and wellbeing insurances to mirror the most recent proof based rehearsals and administrative changes.

2. New Clinical Guidelines: Reconciliation of refreshed clinical rules and conventions for overseeing normal circumstances, guaranteeing medical attendants are outfitted with the latest proposals for patient consideration.

3. Improved Indicative Tools: Presentation of new symptomatic calculations and dynamic devices to help medical caretakers in precisely surveying patient circumstances and deciding suitable mediations.

4. Joining of Proof Based Practices: Combination of the most recent examination discoveries and proof based rehearses into different segments and parts to help inform direction and upgrade patient results.

5. Smoothed out Formatting: Reconsidered organizing and design for further developed comprehensibility and simplicity of route, making it considerably more helpful for medical attendants to rapidly get to fundamental data.

Prologue to New Givers, Master Analyses, and Outside Resources:

In the current year's version, we are happy to invite new givers and master pundits who bring an abundance of information and experience to the handbook. These regarded experts have contributed their bits of knowledge and aptitude to improve the substance and guarantee its significance to contemporary nursing practice.

Also, we have consolidated external assets like internet based data sets, clinical practice rules, and proof based research articles to enhance the data given in the handbook. These assets act as significant enhancements, offering medical caretakers admittance to extra data and points of view to additionally improve their training.

A Speedy Manual for Exploring the Pocket Medication Handbook:

Exploring the Pocket Medication Handbook is presently simpler than any time in recent memory, on account of its easy to use plan and natural design. Here is a speedy manual for distinguishing center segments, going with assets, and exceptional highlights of the current year's version:

1. Center Sections: The handbook is partitioned into unmistakable segments covering a great many points, including pharmacology, diagnostics, sickness the board, and patient consideration. Each part is variety coded for simple distinguishing proof and route.

2. Going with Resources: All through the handbook, you'll track down references to going with assets like internet based data sets, clinical practice rules, and significant exploration articles. These assets give extra setting and backing to the data introduced in the handbook.

3. Novel Features: The current year's release incorporates a few one of a kind highlights intended to improve convenience and work with learning.

These highlights might incorporate speedy reference tables, clinical pearls, mental aides, and contextual analyses to support key ideas and work with understanding.

By really getting to know these center areas, going with assets, and extraordinary elements, you'll be better prepared to use the maximum capacity of the Pocket Medication Handbook and upgrade your nursing practice.

Section Two: Exploring Pocket Medication Ideas: Pragmatic Apparatuses, Computations, and Agendas for Quick, Dependable Independent direction

In the high speed universe of medication, approaching solid apparatuses, estimations, and conventions is fundamental for settling on informed choices rapidly and precisely.

This part will dive into cutting edge computations and details for exact medication dosing and organization, give visual choice guides to quick emergency, investigating, and treatment arranging, and proposition research-based, peer-audited clinical conventions and calculations custom fitted for attendants around the world.

High level Computations and Definitions for Exact Medication Dosing and Organization

Accuracy in drug dosing and organization is foremost to guarantee patient wellbeing and viability. High level estimations and plans furnish medical care experts with the essential devices to decide proper measurements in view of elements like patient weight, age, renal capability, and comorbidities.

Apparatuses and Layouts for Continuous Use

Using apparatuses and layouts intended for continuous use smoothes out the dosing system, diminishing the gamble of blunders and guaranteeing reliable adherence to best practices. These assets might include:

- Weight-Based Dosing Calculators: Calculations and number crunchers custom fitted to patient weight, guaranteeing exact dosing for meds with weight-subordinate pharmacokinetics.

- Renal Dosing Protocols: Rules for changing medication measurements in light of renal capability, limiting the gamble of harmfulness or remedial disappointment in patients with impeded kidney capability.

- Pediatric Dosing Charts: Age-fitting dosing outlines and equations for pediatric patients, representing formative contrasts in drug digestion and leeway.

- **Mixture Rate Calculators:** Instruments for computing implantation rates in light of medication focus, wanted portion, and mixture term, working with exact intravenous drug organization.

- **Pharmacokinetic Models:** High level models for assessing drug focus after some time, streamlining dosing regimens for prescriptions with complex pharmacokinetic profiles.

Visual Choice Guides for Quick, Exact Emergency, Investigating, and Treatment-Arranging

Visual choice guides offer a fast method for surveying patient status, distinguishing expected intricacies, and forming treatment plans custom-made to individual patient requirements and conditions. These guides might take different structures, including flowcharts, calculations, and choice trees.

Altering Care Intends to Fit Individual Patient Necessities and Conditions

Customizing care plans in light of patient-explicit elements is fundamental for streamlining results and upgrading patient fulfillment. Visual choice guides work with this interaction by directing medical care experts through a methodical way to deal with patient evaluation and the executives, considering variables, for example,

- **Clinical Presentations:** Separating between normal clinical introductions and recognizing warnings reminiscent of serious basic pathology.

- **Demonstrative Workup:** Directing the choice of fitting symptomatic tests in view of introducing side effects, clinical discoveries, and hazard factors.

- **Treatment Algorithms:** Giving bit by bit calculations to starting treatment, titrating intercessions, and observing reaction to treatment.

- **Exceptional Populations:** Fitting consideration plans to unique populaces like geriatric patients, pregnant ladies, or patients with complex clinical chronicles.

Research-Based, Companion Surveyed Clinical Conventions and Calculations for Medical caretakers Around the world

Keeping up to date with the most recent proof based clinical conventions and calculations is critical for conveying great consideration. Peer-checked on assets furnish medical attendants with believed rules and suggestions upheld by logical exploration and master agreement.

Guaranteeing Best Practices and Normalization of Care

By sticking to laid out clinical conventions and calculations, medical attendants can guarantee consistency in care conveyance, advance patient security, and enhance asset usage. Key highlights of exploration based clinical conventions include:

- Proof Based Recommendations: Drawing on the most recent exploration discoveries and clinical preliminaries to illuminate best practices in quiet consideration.

- Multidisciplinary Collaboration: Including medical services experts from different claims to fame in convention advancement to guarantee complete and all encompassing patient administration.

- Consistent Quality Improvement: Consolidating input systems and execution measurements to screen convention adherence and distinguish regions for development.

- **Worldwide Applicability:** Fitting conventions to represent provincial varieties in medical services foundation, assets, and illness pervasiveness.

Exploring the intricacies of pocket medication expects admittance to functional devices, estimations, and agendas that empower quick, dependable direction.

High level computations and definitions enable medical care experts to direct prescriptions securely and actually, while visual choice guides work with quick emergency, investigating, and therapy arranging.

Research-based clinical conventions and calculations guarantee normalized care conveyance and advance constant quality improvement, helping attendants overall in their journey to give ideal patient consideration.

Section Three: Health related Crises and Emergency Conventions: Quick Track Independent direction and Activity Taking Apparatuses for Time-Delicate Circumstances

Health related crises request quick and unequivocal activity to advance patient results. This part gives a complete manual for usually experienced health related crises and basic circumstances across different organ frameworks, frames quick track emergency conventions and treatment pathways for normalized nurture drove care the executives, and offers fundamental data on overseeing harmful openings, close suffocating episodes, and injury fatalities.

A Complete Manual for Regularly Experienced Health related Crises and Basic Circumstances

Health related crises can appear across different organ frameworks, introducing difficulties that require brief acknowledgment and mediation. This guide covers many basic circumstances, including:

Cardiopulmonary Crises:

- Intense Myocardial Infarction: Perceiving the signs and side effects of myocardial dead tissue, starting early intercession measures like ibuprofen organization and thrombolytic treatment, and planning care with cardiology associates for emanant revascularization systems.

- Aspiratory Embolism: Recognizing risk factors and clinical signs of pneumonic embolism, carrying out indicative calculations, for example, the Wells score and D-dimer testing, and starting anticoagulant treatment to forestall clots proliferation and embolic intricacies.

Neurological Crises:

- Ischemic Stroke: Surveying stroke seriousness utilizing apparatuses like the NIH Stroke Scale, enacting stroke conventions for opportune neuroimaging and thrombolytic treatment, and giving strong consideration measures to improve neurological recuperation.

- Status Epilepticus: Overseeing delayed seizures with forceful pharmacotherapy, guaranteeing aviation route assurance and cardiovascular adjustment, and distinguishing and treating hidden accelerating factors.

Gastrointestinal Crises:

- Gastrointestinal Bleeding: Separating upper and lower gastrointestinal draining in light of clinical show and hemodynamic soundness, leading earnest endoscopic assessment for source distinguishing proof and hemostasis, and regulating blood items depending on the situation to address coagulopathy and balance out hemodynamics.

Genitourinary Crises:

- Intense Kidney Injury: Perceiving intense kidney injury in light of changes in serum creatinine and pee yield, distinguishing and tending to potential etiologies like hypovolemia, nephrotoxic prescriptions, and obstructive uropathy, and executing renal swap treatment for extreme cases.

Hematologic Crises:

- Spread Intravascular Coagulation (DIC): Recognizing DISC in the setting of sepsis, injury, or threat, adjusting basic triggers while overseeing coagulopathy with blood items and anticoagulant treatment, and intently checking for confusions like draining and organ brokenness.

Endocrine Crises:

- Diabetic Ketoacidosis (DKA): Perceiving DKA in patients with diabetes mellitus in light of hyperglycemia, ketosis, and metabolic acidosis, starting forceful liquid revival and insulin treatment, and checking for electrolyte aggravations and cerebral edema.

Quick Track Emergency Conventions and Treatment Pathways

Proficient emergency conventions and treatment pathways are fundamental for advancing asset use and smoothing out care conveyance in crisis settings. Acknowledged, rehearsed, and explored upheld approaches for nurture drove emergency and mind the executives include:

Emergency Calculations:

- Manchester Emergency System: Using a variety coded calculation to focus on persistent evaluation and intercession in light of the seriousness of introducing side effects and physiological boundaries.

- **Crisis Seriousness List (ESI):** Carrying out a five-level emergency calculation to classify patients as per sharpness level, taking into consideration fast ID of high-risk cases requiring quick mediation.

Treatment Pathways:

- **Sepsis Bundle:** Following proof based conventions for the early acknowledgment and the board of sepsis, including brief inception of antimicrobials, liquid revival, and vasopressor treatment to forestall movement to septic shock.

- **Injury Revival Protocol:** Complying with normalized injury calculations, for example, High level Injury Life Backing (ATLS) or Prehospital Injury Life Backing (PHTLS) rules to guarantee methodical evaluation and treatment of harmed patients, with an emphasis on essential review, revival, and conclusive consideration.

A Manual for Overseeing Ordinarily Experienced Harmful Openings, Close Suffocating, and Injury Fatalities

Attendants in crisis, basic consideration, and injury settings should be prepared to deal with different testing situations, including poisonous openings, close suffocating occurrences, and injury fatalities. Fundamental data for these circumstances incorporates:

Poisonous Openings:

- **Poison Control Resources:** Using poison control focuses and online information bases to distinguish poisons, evaluate harmfulness levels, and decide suitable administration procedures, like sterilization, remedy organization, and strong consideration.

Close Suffocating Occurrences:

- **Prompt Resuscitation:** Starting cardiopulmonary revival (CPR) and high level life support estimates in case of close suffocating, including aviation route the executives, oxygenation, and ventilation, trailed by quick exchange to a clinical office for additional assessment and the board.

Injury Fatalities:

- **Demise Notification:** Giving empathetic and delicate correspondence while conveying insight about a horrendous passing to relatives, offering backing and assets for adapting to despondency and misfortune.

Health related crises request quick and definitive activity, requiring medical services experts to be knowledgeable in perceiving basic circumstances, executing quick track emergency conventions, and overseeing testing situations like poisonous openings, close suffocating episodes, and injury fatalities.

By sticking to normalized conventions and drawing on proof based rehearsals, attendants can upgrade patient results and give great consideration in time-delicate circumstances.

Explore another similar amazing book titled

Assist Me To Quit Thinking

Your Blueprint to Emotional Mastery and a Life of Tranquility

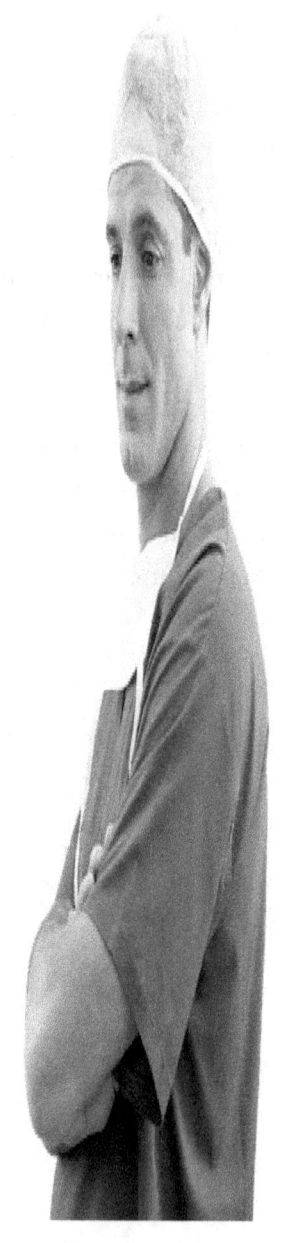

Section Four: Illness Explicit Nursing Care: Viable, Quick Reference Advisers for Key Monographs, Sickness Cycles, and Nursing Mediations

Illness explicit nursing care requires a profound comprehension of different sicknesses, conditions, and methodology experienced in present day nursing practice.

This part gives a far reaching manual for normal infections, conditions, and systems, frames quick track sickness explicit nursing care plans, studios, and instructing/learning devices, and offers a speedy manual for overseeing regularly experienced ongoing illnesses, conditions, and methods.

A Thorough Manual for Normal Sicknesses, Conditions, and Methods Experienced in Present day Nursing Practice

Attendants experience a different scope of sicknesses, conditions, and methods in their day to day practice, each requiring a fitted way to deal with nursing care. This thorough aide covers a wide cluster of clinical issues, including:

Respiratory Issues:

- **Asthma and COPD:** Overseeing constant respiratory circumstances portrayed via aviation route irritation and wind stream impediment, remembering patient instruction for inhaler methods, checking for intensifications, and carrying out customized activity plans.

Cardiovascular Circumstances:

- **Congestive Cardiovascular breakdown (CHF):** Furnishing care for patients with weakened cardiovascular capability, including observing liquid equilibrium, directing diuretics and vasodilators, and instructing patients on salt and liquid limitation.

- **Myocardial Localized necrosis (MI):** Overseeing intense coronary disorder with an emphasis on early acknowledgment, torment the board, oxygen treatment, and organization of antiplatelet and anticoagulant drugs.

Irresistible Illnesses:

- **Sepsis:** Perceiving the signs and side effects of foundational incendiary reaction condition (SIRS) and sepsis, starting early objective coordinated treatment, and checking for entanglements like organ brokenness and septic shock.

- **Aspiratory Embolism (PE):** Evaluating risk factors and clinical signs of PE, executing anticoagulant treatment, and checking for hemodynamic insecurity and respiratory split the difference.

Neurological Problems:

- **Stroke:** Giving intense consideration to patients with ischemic or hemorrhagic stroke, including thrombolytic treatment, neuroprotective measures, and restoration intercessions to upgrade useful recuperation.

Renal Brokenness:

- **Renal Failure:** Overseeing intricacies of intense and persistent renal disappointment, including electrolyte lopsided characteristics, liquid over-burden, and metabolic acidosis, and working together with the medical care group to start renal substitution treatment on a case by case basis.

Psychological wellness Issues:

- Discouragement and Nervousness Disorders: Supporting patients with temperament and nervousness problems through helpful correspondence, conduct intercessions, and pharmacological administration, while advancing taking care of oneself and survival techniques.

Irresistible Circumstances:

- Pneumonia and Cellulitis: Evaluating and overseeing bacterial diseases like pneumonia and cellulitis, including anti-infection treatment, strong consideration, and checking for treatment reaction and entanglements.

Urological Conditions:

- Urinary Parcel Diseases (UTIs): Recognizing risk factors and clinical appearances of UTIs, acquiring suitable pee societies, and directing antimicrobial treatment in view of responsiveness results.

Vascular Problems:

- Profound Vein Apoplexy (DVT): Perceiving risk factors and clinical appearances of DVT, carrying out anticoagulant treatment to forestall blood clot engendering and embolic complexities, and advancing ambulation and pressure treatment.

Quick Track Illness Explicit Nursing Care Plans, Studios, and Educating/Learning Apparatuses

Making effective, proof based, and individualized care plans is fundamental for tending to the complex and comorbid needs of patients with different infections and conditions.

Quick track sickness explicit nursing care plans, studios, and educating/learning devices give viable direction and assets to attendants in conveying excellent consideration.

Care Arranging:

- Appraisal and Diagnosis: Leading complete evaluations to distinguish patient requirements, qualities, and inclinations, and figuring out nursing analysis in view of information examination and clinical judgment.

- Objective Setting and Mediation Planning: Teaming up with patients and interdisciplinary colleagues to lay out sensible objectives and foster proof based intercessions to address recognized nursing, analyze and accomplish wanted results.

- Assessment and Documentation: Checking patient reactions to medications, assessing progress towards objectives, and reporting evaluation discoveries, intercessions, and results in an ideal and precise way.

Studios and Educating/Learning Instruments:

- Reenactment Based Training: Taking part in involved reproductions to rehearse clinical abilities, decisive reasoning, and dynamic in a controlled climate, considering experiential mastering and expertise securing.

- Contextual investigations and Issue Based Learning: Dissecting case situations and participating in critical thinking exercises to apply hypothetical information to true nursing work, cultivating dynamic acquiring and clinical thinking abilities.

- **Instructive Resources:** Getting to online modules, course readings, clinical rules, and other instructive materials to improve comprehension of sickness processes, nursing intercessions, and proof based practice rules.

A Fast Manual for Overseeing Normally Experienced Persistent Illnesses, Conditions, and Systems

Persistent illnesses present continuous difficulties for medical caretakers, requiring a diverse way to deal with the executives and care. This fast aide offers pragmatic methodologies for overseeing generally experienced ongoing infections, conditions, and systems, including:

Hypertension and Diabetes:

- **Hypertension:** Carrying out way of life changes, pharmacological treatment, and normal checking to control circulatory strain and decrease cardiovascular gamble.

- **Diabetes Mellitus:** Giving instruction on glucose observing, insulin organization, dietary administration, and foot care to advance glycemic control and forestall difficulties.

Metabolic and Endocrine Issues:

- **Obesity:** Offering guidance on nourishment, active work, and changing on a surface level strategies to help weight reduction and further develop generally speaking wellbeing results.

- **Osteoporosis:** Instructing patients on calcium and vitamin D supplementation, fall anticipation techniques, and pharmacological intercessions to forestall breaks and keep up with bone wellbeing.

- **Thyroid Disorders:** Observing thyroid capability tests, changing thyroid chemical substitution treatment depending on the situation, and teaching patients on signs and side effects of hypo-and hyperthyroidism.

Respiratory Circumstances:

- **Asthma and COPD:** Showing inhaler strategies, executing smoking end intercessions, and giving pneumonic restoration to upgrade respiratory capability and personal satisfaction.

Cardiovascular Infections:

- **Congestive Cardiovascular breakdown (CHF) and Coronary Supply route Illness (CAD):**

Overseeing side effects through medicine adherence, dietary sodium limitation, and liquid administration, and elevating adherence to heart restoration programs for optional counteraction.

Gastrointestinal Problems:

- Peevish Inside Disorder (IBS): Suggesting dietary alterations, stress the board strategies, and pharmacological treatments to mitigate side effects and work on personal satisfaction.

Oncological Medical procedure and Therapies:

- Malignant growth Medical procedure and Chemotherapy: Supporting patients through the perioperative period, overseeing therapy related secondary effects, and offering profound help and side effects to the board all through the malignant growth venture.

Constant Agony The executives:

- Torment Appraisal and Multimodal Therapy: Leading far reaching torment appraisals, executing individualized torment the executives plans consolidating pharmacological and non-pharmacological intercessions, and advancing patient independence and self-administration systems.

Emotional wellness Problems:

- Uneasiness, Despondency, and Insane Disorders: Teaming up with mental suppliers to improve prescription administration, giving psychoeducation and strong advising, and interfacing patients with local area assets for progressing support.

Illness explicit nursing care requires a profound comprehension of different sicknesses, conditions, and systems experienced in current nursing practice. By using extensive aides, quick track care plans, studios, and instructing/learning devices, medical attendants can effectively convey proof based and individualized care to patients with complex and comorbid needs. Also, fast aides offer useful techniques for overseeing regularly experienced persistent

infections, conditions, and methodology, engaging attendants to enhance patient results and work on personal satisfaction.

Section Five: Working Situations and Reproductions: Specialist Checked Difficulties, Circumstances, and Proof Based Reactions for Attendants

Exploring job situations gives a heap of difficulties, going from moral predicaments to fierce experiences and high-stress circumstances.

This part gives a manual for dealing with moral and expert problems, quick track reactions and conventions for managing requesting people, and methodologies for keeping up with top notch nursing care, sympathy, and correspondence in speedy settings.

A Manual for Exploring Moral and Expert Problems

Moral and expert quandaries are an inescapable part of nursing work, expecting medical attendants to explore complex circumstances while maintaining moral guidelines and lawful commitments. Quick track ways to deal with independent direction include:

Moral Dynamic Structures:

- **Standards Based Approach:** Applying moral standards like independence, value, non-wrathfulness, and equity to examine difficulties and guide dynamics as per moral thinking.

- **Moral Dynamic Models:** Using organized structures, for example, the Four-Part Model (ACNM) or the Moral Dynamic System (EDMF) to efficiently survey moral issues, distinguish choices, and assess possible results.

Proficient Norms and Rules:

- **Nursing Codes of Ethics:** Sticking to laid out implicit sets of rules like the American Medical attendants Affiliation (ANA) Overarching set of principles for Medical caretakers, which gives direction on moral obligations, proficient lead, and support for patients' privileges.

- **Legitimate Considerations:** Finding out more about important regulations, guidelines, and institutional approaches administering nursing work, guaranteeing consistency with legitimate necessities and staying away from proficient responsibility.

Quick Track Reactions and Conventions for Experiencing Fierce and Requesting People

Experiences with fierce or requesting patients, relatives, and partners can introduce difficulties to keeping up with impressive skill and guaranteeing patient security. Quick track reactions and conventions include:

De-acceleration Strategies:

- **Dynamic Listening:** Recognizing the singular's interests and feelings, showing compassion, and approving their viewpoint to lay out affinity and stop pressure.

- **Compromise Skills: Utilizing** self-assured correspondence procedures, for example, "I" proclamations and reexamining, to address clashes productively and cooperatively.

Defining Limits:

- Decisive Communication: Obviously articulating assumptions, cutoff points, and results in a deferential way, declaring one's freedoms as well as expectations while keeping up with impressive skill.

- Security Protocols: Carrying out institutional conventions for overseeing forceful ways of behaving, including the utilization of deceleration groups, security staff, or emergency mediation techniques.

A Manual for Incredible Days, Movements, and Evenings: Specialist Checked Approaches for Keeping up with Top notch Nursing Care, Sympathy, and Correspondence

Keeping up with great nursing care, sympathy, and correspondence is fundamental for advancing positive patient results and encouraging a steady workplace. Professional confirmed approaches include:

Taking care of oneself Methodologies:

- Stress The board Techniques: Consolidating pressure decreases exercises like care, contemplation, profound breathing activities, or actual activity into everyday schedules to improve versatility and adapting abilities.

- Work-Life Balance: Focusing on private time, side interests, and connections beyond work to forestall burnout and keep up with close to home prosperity.

Group Joint effort:

- Interdisciplinary Collaboration: Drawing in with partners from various medical services disciplines to advance facilitated care, share information and aptitude, and enhance patient results.

- Peer Backing Networks: Laying out peer encouraging groups of people or mentorship projects to offer close to home help, share encounters, and cultivate proficient development and improvement.

Relational abilities:

- Compelling Correspondence Strategies: Rehearsing clear, brief, and compassionate correspondence with patients, families, and associates, using undivided attention, restorative correspondence procedures, and unconditional addressing to improve understanding and compatibility.

- Compromise and Feedback: Tending to clashes and giving useful criticism in a conscious and non-critical way, advancing a culture of open correspondence, shared regard, and persistent improvement.

On the job situations and reenactments present medical caretakers with various difficulties, from moral problems to angry experiences and high-stress circumstances.

By utilizing quick track ways to deal with independent direction, de-acceleration methods, and taking care of oneself procedures, medical attendants can explore these situations with incredible skill, empathy, and versatility.

Powerful correspondence, joint effort, and adherence to proficient norms are vital to keeping up with top notch nursing care and advancing positive patient results in high speed medical services settings.

Section Six: Overseeing Pressure, Burnout, and Prosperity: Functional Instruments, Strategies, and Strategies for Advancing Taking care of oneself and Balance between serious and fun activities

Overseeing pressure, forestalling burnout, and advancing prosperity are fundamental parts of keeping a solid and satisfying nursing vocation.

This part offers viable instruments, procedures, and strategies for creating compelling pressure on the executives systems, recognizing and overseeing work environment stressors, and making customized taking care of oneself practices to advance long haul prosperity, strength, and individual fulfillment.

A Fast Manual for Making a Compelling Pressure The board Methodology

Making a powerful pressure the executives technique is fundamental for medical caretakers to keep up with their prosperity and strength in requesting medical services conditions. Functional apparatuses, strategies, and strategies include:

Stress Appraisal:

- **Distinguishing Stressors**: Perceiving normal stressors in the work environment, for example, high responsibility, time pressure, clashes with associates, and profound requests of patient consideration.

- **Self-Reflection:** Pondering individual pressure triggers, strategies for dealing with especially difficult times, and regions for development in overseeing pressure successfully.

Stress-Decrease Strategies:

- **Care and Meditation:** Rehearsing care based methods, like profound breathing activities, moderate muscle unwinding, and directed reflection, to advance unwinding and stress decrease.

- Actual Activity: Integrating customary activity into day to day schedules, like strolling, running, yoga, or dance, to deliver strain, further develop mind-set, and upgrade generally speaking prosperity.

Time Usage Systems:

- Prioritization: Distinguishing high-need assignments and distributing time and assets appropriately to limit overpower and expand efficiency.

- Setting Boundaries: Laying out clear limits among work and individual life, including booking normal breaks, restricting additional time, and assigning errands when important.

A Manual for Recognizing and Overseeing Working environment Stressors and High-Chance Situations

Recognizing and overseeing working environment stressors and high-risk situations are significant for forestalling burnout and advancing a solid workplace. Expert checked reactions include:

Stressor Recognizable proof:

- **Natural Stressors:** Surveying actual variables in the workplace, like clamor, lighting, temperature, and ergonomic plan, and making acclimations to improve solace and diminish pressure.

- **Relational Stressors:** Tending to clashes with associates, correspondence breakdowns, and various leveled pressures through open discourse, compromise procedures, and collaboration systems.

High-Chance Situation The board:

- **Basic Episode Debriefing:** Working with organized interviewing meetings following basic episodes or horrible accidents to handle feelings, share encounters, and advance mental prosperity among colleagues.

- **Security Protocols:** Executing security measures and conventions to alleviate takes a chance in high-stress situations, like patient hostility, health related crises, or work environment savagery.

A Manual for Making Customized Taking care of oneself Practices

Making customized taking care of oneself practices is fundamental for attendants to support their prosperity, flexibility, and occupation fulfillment over the long haul. Professional checked devices, methods, and strategies include:

Taking care of oneself Appraisal:

- Self-Reflection: Participating in thoughtfulness to distinguish individual requirements, values, qualities, and regions for development in advancing taking care of oneself and prosperity.

- Self-Compassion: Developing a merciful mentality towards oneself, recognizing impediments, and rehearsing taking care of oneself without responsibility or judgment.

Taking care of oneself Practices:

- Solid Way of life Habits: Focusing on exercises that advance actual wellbeing, like nutritious eating, normal activity, satisfactory rest, and hydration, to help by and large prosperity.

- Relaxation and Recreation: Participating in charming leisure activities, interests, and recreation exercises beyond work to cultivate unwinding, imagination, and individual satisfaction.

Social Encouraging groups of people:

- **Peer Support:** Interfacing with partners, companions, and relatives for everyday reassurance, consolation, and social connection, encouraging a feeling of having a place and local area.

- **Proficient Support:** Searching out mentorship, management, or directing administrations to address proficient difficulties, improve adapting abilities, and advance profession fulfillment.

Overseeing pressure, forestalling burnout, and advancing prosperity are fundamental parts of keeping a solid and satisfying nursing vocation.

By creating viable pressure on the executives systems, recognizing and overseeing working environment stressors, and developing customized taking care of oneself practices, attendants can support their prosperity, strength, and occupation fulfillment over the long haul.

Focusing on taking care of oneself advantages individual attendants as well as adds to a positive workplace and improves patient consideration results.

Section Seven: Research-Based Efficient and Professional success Tips: Expert Confirmed Methodologies for Utilizing the Lippincott Pocket Medication Handbook for Attendants

The Lippincott Pocket Medication Handbook for Medical Caretakers is a significant asset for medical caretakers, offering speedy admittance to fundamental data for clinical work on, proceeding with schooling, and professional success.

This part gives commonsense tips and procedures to utilizing this handbook to create vocation propelling introductions, improve nursing practice, and interface with friends, coaches, and industry pioneers.

A Manual for Creating One of a kind, Vocation Propelling Introductions, Studios, Classes, and Instructional meetings

Creating connections with useful introductions, studios, classes, and instructional meetings is a critical expertise for propelling your nursing profession. Professional confirmed devices, strategies, and strategies include:

Show Plan:

- Clear Objectives: Characterize clear goals and learning results for your show, guaranteeing arrangement with the requirements and interests of your crowd.

- Drawing in Content: Consolidate media components, contextual investigations, intelligent activities, and genuine guides to enthrall your crowd and upgrade learning viability.

Conveyance Procedures:

- Compelling Communication: Practice viable relational abilities, like certain talking, undivided attention, and drawing in narrating, to associate with your crowd and pass on key messages really.

- Intuitive Engagement: Support crowd interest through interactive discussions, bunch conversations, and involved exercises, cultivating dynamic learning and information maintenance.

A Manual for Utilizing the Lippincott Pocket Medication Handbook for Medical attendants as a Training Enhancer, Abilities Developer, and Proceeding with Schooling Asset

The Lippincott Pocket Medication Handbook for Attendants fills in as a flexible device for improving nursing work on, building abilities, and proceeding with training. Reasonable ways to use this asset include:

Clinical Reference:

- **Fast Admittance to Information:** Use the handbook's compact configuration and coordinated format to rapidly get to fundamental data on meds, symptomatic tests, clinical rules, and nursing techniques.

- **Proof Based Practice:** Utilize the handbook to keep up- to-date with proof based practice rules, integrating the most recent exploration discoveries and best practices into your clinical independent direction.

Abilities Upgrade:

- System Guidance: Allude to the handbook for bit by bit direction on performing normal nursing methodology, like drug organization, wound care, and venipuncture, guaranteeing precision and adherence to best practices.

- Decisive Reasoning Exercises: Participate in decisive reasoning activities and contextual analyses given in the handbook to improve your clinical thinking abilities and upgrade critical abilities to think.

Proceeding with Schooling:

- Independent Learning: Make the most of the handbook's thorough substance to seek after independent learning, open doors, investigate areas of premium, extend your insight base, and proceed with instruction credits.

- Proficient Development: Utilize the handbook as an instrument for proficient turn of events, defining learning objectives, following advancement, and considering your training to distinguish regions for development and improvement.

A Manual for Interfacing with Companions, Tutors, and Industry Pioneers

Building an expert organization is fundamental for propelling your nursing vocation and remaining informed about arising patterns and potential open doors. Specialist checked devices and strategies for interfacing with friends, tutors, and industry pioneers include:

Organizing Techniques:

- Proficient Associations: Join nursing associations and expert affiliations pertinent to your forte or area of interest, taking part in gatherings, meetings, and online discussions to connect with friends and pioneers in the field.

- Virtual Entertainment Platforms: Use virtual entertainment stages like LinkedIn, Twitter, and expert nursing gatherings to associate with partners, share bits of knowledge, and participate in conversations on important subjects.

Mentorship and Direction:

- **Looking for Mentorship:** Distinguish experienced medical attendants, teachers, or pioneers in your association or local area who can give mentorship, direction, and vocation exhortation to help your expert development and advancement.

- **Peer Backing Groups:** Structure or join peer support gatherings or mentorship circles with individual medical caretakers, offering common consolation, responsibility, and information sharing open doors.

Utilizing the Lippincott Pocket Medication Handbook for Attendants and carrying out research-based methodologies can altogether upgrade your nursing practice, advance your vocation, and work with proficient development and improvement.

By creating drawings in introductions, using the handbook as a training enhancer and proceeding with schooling assets, and effectively connecting with companions, tutors, and industry pioneers, you can situate yourself for progress and make significant commitments to the nursing calling.

Section Eight: Interactive media Enhancements and Assets: Intuitive Devices, Introductions, Recordings, and Studios for Improving Nursing Experts' Abilities and Information

Mixed media enhancements and assets assume an urgent part in improving nursing experts' abilities, information, and professional success valuable open doors.

This part gives an exhaustive manual for quick track, on-office proceeding with training assets, using interactive media supplements for upgrading patient consideration and local area instruction, and utilizing these assets for individual abilities improvement, initiative potential, and practice-incorporation endeavors.

A Manual for Quick Track, On-Office Proceeding with Training Assets

Quick track, on-office proceeding with instruction assets offer helpful and available ways for nursing experts to improve their abilities, information, and professional success open doors. Expert checked apparatuses, procedures, and strategies include:

Web based Learning Stages:

- Proceeding with Instruction Modules: Getting to online courses, online courses, and self-guided modules presented by trustworthy associations and instructive establishments to acquire proceeding with training credits and keep up to date with the most recent advancements in nursing practice.

- Virtual Conferences: Partaking in virtual meetings and conferences zeroed in on nursing strengths, arising patterns, and proof based works on, considering organizing amazing open doors and information trade with specialists in the field.

Digital recordings and Sound Assets:

- Instructive Podcasts: Paying attention to nursing-centered digital broadcasts covering many points, from clinical updates and contextual investigations to administration advancement and expert development, during drives or margin time to enhance learning and remain informed.

- Book recordings and Lectures: Getting to book recordings and recorded addresses on nursing subjects of interest, giving adaptability to learning in a hurry and building up key ideas through continued tuning in.

A Manual for Utilizing Interactive media Enhancements and Assets for Upgrading Patient Consideration, People group Schooling, and Practice-Contact Endeavors

Media enhancements and assets offer important devices for improving patient consideration, local area training, and practice contact endeavors. Down to earth tips for usage include:

Patient Schooling Materials:

- Intuitive Recordings and Demonstrations: Using mixed media assets to make intuitive recordings and shows on themes like prescription organization, wound care, and self-administration strategies, upgrading patient getting it and adherence to treatment plans.

- Advanced Wellbeing Tools: Coordinating computerized wellbeing devices and applications into patient training endeavors, for example, portable applications for prescription updates, side effect following, and virtual conferences, to engage patients in dealing with their wellbeing and advancing taking care of oneself.

Local area Effort Projects:

- Instructive Studios and Seminars: Putting together instructive studios and classes for local area individuals on preventive well being measures, constant sickness the executives, and solid way of life ways of behaving, encouraging wellbeing education and advancing health inside the local area.

- Wellbeing Fair Exhibits: Setting up intelligent shows and enlightening corners at wellbeing fairs and local area occasions to scatter proof based wellbeing data, direct wellbeing screenings, and associate local area individuals with neighborhood medical care assets and administrations.

Practice Contact Drives:

- Interactive media Introductions and Reports: Making interactive media introductions and reports to feature practice accomplishments, quality improvement drives, and patient results to partners, including clinic heads, policymakers, and financing organizations, to accumulate backing and acknowledgment for nursing drives.

- Virtual Visits and Telehealth Demonstrations: Offering virtual voyages through medical services offices and exhibitions of telehealth administrations to forthcoming patients, local area associations, and alluding suppliers, featuring mechanical advancements and admittance to mind choices.

A Manual for Using Sight and sound Enhancements and Assets for Upgrading Individual Abilities, Initiative Potential, and Practice-Joining Endeavors

Sight and sound enhancements and assets are important devices for improving individual abilities, administration potential, and practice-reconciliation endeavors among nursing experts. Systems for use include:

Individual Abilities Improvement:

- Online Expertise building Courses: Signing up for online courses and studios zeroed in on self-awareness regions like relational abilities, using time effectively, flexibility, and the capacity to appreciate anyone on a deeper level, to improve viability in both expert and individual spaces.

- Self-evaluation Tools: Utilizing mixed media assets, for example, self-evaluation tests and intuitive activities to distinguish qualities, regions for development, and learning inclinations, working with designated ability advancement and mindfulness.

Authority Advancement:

- Initiative Preparation Modules: Taking part in administration advancement projects and modules presented through web-based stages or expert associations, zeroing in on authority styles, group building, compromise, and vital preparation, to get ready for influential positions inside the nursing calling.

- Mentorship and Coaching: Searching out mentorship and training open doors with experienced nursing pioneers or chief mentors to get direction, criticism, and backing in exploring professional success and administration challenges.

Practice-Coordination Endeavors:

- **Multidisciplinary Cooperation Tools:** Utilizing sight and sound assets to work with correspondence and cooperation among multidisciplinary medical services groups, for example, virtual joint effort stages, shared dynamic instruments, and video chatting programming, to further develop coordination of care and patient results.

- **Quality Improvement Initiatives:** Using mixed media assets to report and spread discoveries from quality improvement projects, clinical examination studies, and proof based practice drives inside medical care associations, advancing practice joining and information interpretation.

Sight and sound enhancements and assets offer assorted open doors for improving nursing experts' abilities, information, and professional success possibilities.

By utilizing quick track, on-office proceeding with training assets, using media instruments for patient consideration and local area schooling, and outfitting these assets for individual abilities improvement, initiative potential, and practice-coordination endeavors, medical attendants can raise their training and make significant commitments to medical services conveyance and results.

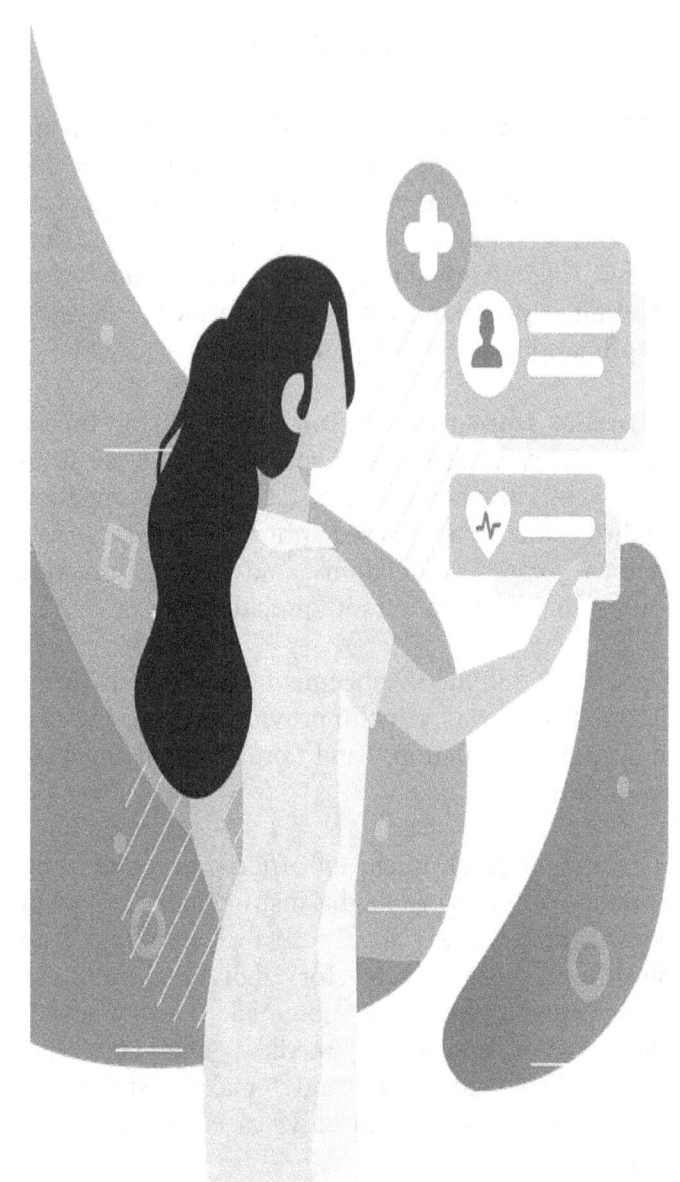

Epilog: A Time of Learning,

Development, and Headway for Nursing Experts Around the world

As we close this excursion, we consider the extraordinary encounters and important illustrations advanced by nursing experts around the world. From humble perusers to certain specialists, from excited students to visionary pioneers, this previous year has been a time of significant development and headway in the nursing calling.

In this epilogue, we offer experiences into creating compelling learning pathways, administration projects, and proceeding with schooling objectives, alongside private tributes and ways to use the Lippincott Pocket Medication Handbook for Medical attendants as a manual for individual and expert development and accomplishment.

Pondering the Extraordinary Excursion

For the majority of nursing experts, the previous year has been set apart by huge achievements and extraordinary encounters. As we changed from perusers to experts, we embraced the difficulties and open doors that came our direction, utilizing our insight and abilities to have a beneficial outcome on quiet consideration and medical services results.

From dominating clinical methodology to exploring moral predicaments, from encouraging cooperation and joint effort to driving quality improvement drives, we have filled in certainty and skill, embracing our jobs as confided in parental figures and backers for our patients.

A Manual for Making Viable Learning Pathways and Initiative Tasks

Creating powerful learning pathways and administration projects is fundamental for nursing experts trying to propel their professions and make significant commitments to their training settings.

By laying out customized objectives, distinguishing regions for development, and creating activity plans for accomplishment, medical caretakers can diagram a course for progress and nonstop improvement. Key methodologies include:

- **Objective Setting:** Characterize clear and attainable learning targets, initiative objectives, and expert advancement targets, adjusting them to hierarchical needs and individual interests.

- Ability Development: Distinguish valuable open doors for expertise upgrade and information obtaining through proper instruction, active preparation, mentorship, and independent learning drives.

- Project Management: Plan and execute authority projects, quality improvement drives, and examination tries utilizing organized strategies and proof based works on, teaming up with interdisciplinary groups and partners to accomplish wanted results.

- Assessment and Reflection: Routinely evaluate progress towards objectives, consider encounters and illustrations learned, and change methodologies depending on the situation to remain focused and boost adequacy.

Individual Tributes, Tips, and Deceives for Utilizing the Lippincott Pocket Medication Handbook for Attendants

The Lippincott Pocket Medication Handbook for Attendants has been an imperative sidekick on our excursion of individual and expert development.

Here, nursing experts share their own tributes, tips, and deceives for boosting the utility of this significant asset:

- **Efficiency:** " The pocket handbook has been a lifeline during occupied shifts. Its succinct organization and coordinated format make it simple to find fundamental data rapidly, permitting me to give ideal and precise consideration to my patients."

- **Accuracy:** " I value the handbook's proof based content and forward-thinking rules, which have assisted me with pursuing informed clinical choices and guarantee the security and prosperity of my patients."

- **Versatility:** " Whether I'm at the bedside, in the study hall, or going to a gathering, the pocket handbook is dependably reachable. Its conservative size and extensive inclusion make it a flexible instrument for all parts of nursing practice."

- **Proceeding with Education:** " As a deep rooted student, I esteem the handbook's job in supporting my proceeding with schooling endeavors. Its references to extra assets and online materials have directed me in investigating new subjects and growing my insight base."

- **Confidence:** " Having the pocket handbook close by gives me trust in my capacities as an attendant. It fills in as a confided in friend, offering consolation and direction in testing circumstances."

As we think back on the previous year of learning, development, and headway, we are helped to remember the flexibility, devotion, and energy that characterize the nursing calling.

From embracing new difficulties to quickly taking advantage of chances for proficient turn of events, nursing experts overall have shown their obligation to greatness and their immovable commitment to the prosperity of their patients.

 As we proceed with our process forward, let us convey forward the examples taken in, the abilities obtained, and the connections manufactured, knowing that together, we can have an effect in the existence of those we serve.

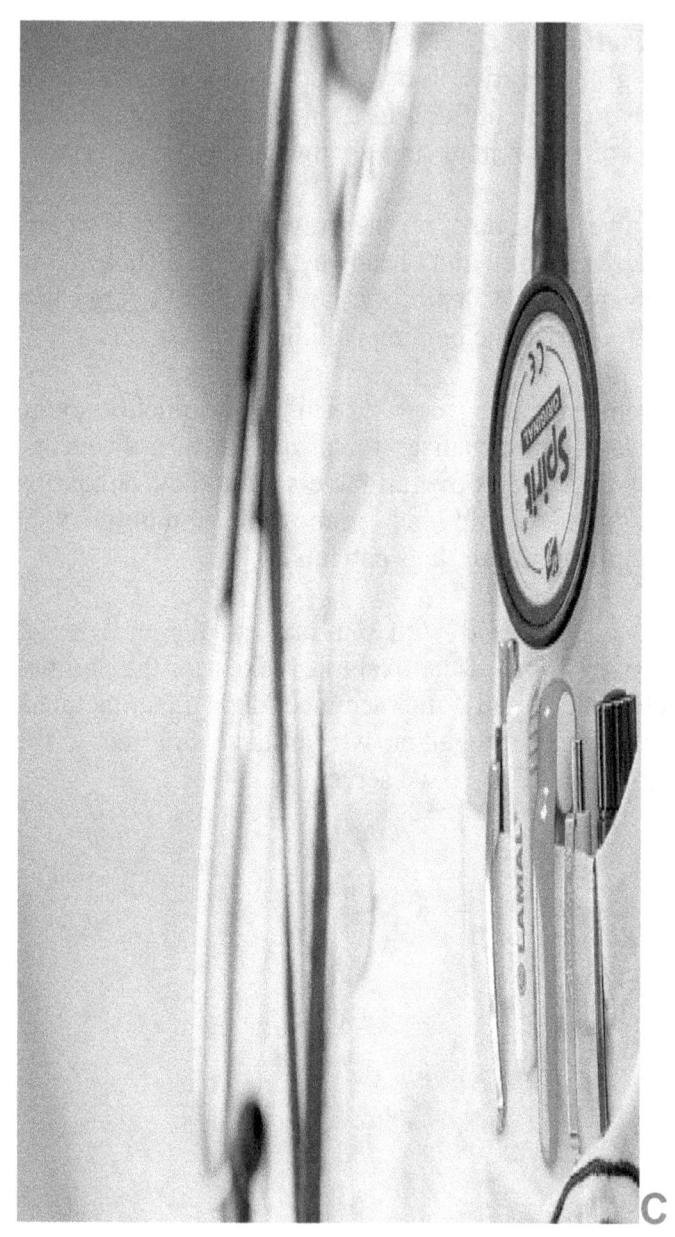

C

onclusion: A Tradition of Greatness in Nursing Care and Schooling

In finishing up our investigation of powerful, enabling, and quick track learning pathways for nursing experts around the world, we ponder the tradition of greatness in nursing care and schooling that has been developed through this book.

From dominating fundamental clinical abilities to embracing initiative open doors, from utilizing creative assets to encouraging a culture of long lasting getting the hang of, nursing experts have exhibited their obligation to conveying excellent consideration and propelling the nursing calling.

In this end, we feature key action items and experiences acquired from our excursion together, praising the aggregate accomplishments and commitments of nursing experts around the world.

Embracing a Culture of Greatness

All through this book, we have underscored the significance of embracing a culture of greatness in nursing care and schooling. Nursing experts significantly affect the wellbeing and prosperity of people, families, and networks, and it is through a guarantee to greatness that we can convey the best quality of care to those we serve.

By consistently taking a stab at progress, searching out potential open doors for development, and maintaining the upsides of impressive skill, sympathy, and respectability, nursing experts can leave an enduring tradition of greatness in their training settings and then some.

Engaging Learning Pathways

Engaging learning pathways are fundamental for nursing experts trying to improve their abilities, information, and profession valuable open doors. By adopting a proactive strategy to proficient turn of events, medical caretakers can graph their own course for progress and satisfaction in their vocations.

From chasing after cutting edge confirmations and specialty preparing to participating in interdisciplinary coordinated efforts and authority improvement drives, there are endless roads for development and progression in the nursing calling. By bridging the force of independent learning, mentorship, and consistent criticism, nursing experts can open their maximum capacity and make significant commitments to their training settings and the more extensive medical care local area.

Quick Track Systems for Progress

In the present quick moving medical care climate, nursing experts need admittance to quick track techniques for progress. This book has given viable devices, strategies, and strategies for exploring the intricacies of present day nursing practice, from efficient estimations and dynamic guides to mixed media enhancements and assets.

By utilizing creative advances, proof based rehearsals, and interdisciplinary coordinated efforts, nursing experts can smooth out their work processes, upgrade patient results, and drive positive change in their training settings.

By embracing an outlook of nimbleness, versatility, and development, nursing experts can flourish in unique medical services conditions and lead the way towards a more promising time to come for nursing care and schooling.

A Source of inspiration

As we finish up our investigation of viable, engaging, and quick track learning pathways for nursing experts around the world, we issue a source of inspiration for all nursing experts to proceed with their excursion of development, learning, and greatness.

By embracing the standards of long lasting learning, impressive skill, and coordinated effort, nursing experts can have a significant effect on the existence of their patients and the networks they serve.

Allow us to subscribe to the quest for greatness in nursing care and training, realizing that our aggregate endeavors will shape the eventual fate of medical services and rouse ages of nursing experts to come.

All things considered, we praise the tradition of greatness in nursing care and schooling that has been developed through this book.

From engaging learning pathways to quick track procedures for progress, nursing experts overall have shown their obligation to greatness and advancement in their training. As we proceed with our process forward, let us convey forward the examples taken in, the abilities obtained, and the connections produced, knowing that together, we can make a significant and enduring effect on the wellbeing and prosperity of people and networks all over the planet.

Much obliged to you for going along with us on this excursion, and may we keep on taking a stab at greatness in all that we do.

Happy reading

Thank you for reading please kindly drop your comments and for more books by me kindly visit my
Author Center page

stay safe

www.ingramcontent.com/pod-product-compliance
Lightning Source LLC
Chambersburg PA
CBHW070945290526
45795CB00005B/1644